AN ULTIMATE GUIDE TO PLASTIC AND RECONSTRUCTIVE SURGERY

I0454546

Exploring History, Techniques, Types, Complications from the Good, the Bad and the Ugly of Plastic Surgery

Micheal Holmes

TABLE OF CONTENTS

CHAPTER 7

ETHICAL AND SOCIETAL CONSIDERATIONS IN PLASTIC SURGERY

CHAPTER 8

RISKS AND COMPLICATIONS IN PLASTIC SURGERY

CHAPTER 9

PERSONAL STORIES AND INTERVIEWS

CHAPTER 10

THE FUTURE OF PLASTIC SURGERY

CHAPTER 11

CONCLUSION

CHAPTER 1

INTRODUCTION TO PLASTIC SURGERY

Welcome to the fascinating world of plastic surgery, a field that combines art and science to alter, restore, or enhance physical appearance. This book aims to demystify the complex and often misunderstood world of plastic surgery, providing insights into its history, techniques, and the impact it has on individuals and society.

At its core, **Plastic Surgery** is a medical specialty focused on the correction or restoration of form and function. While the term often conjures images of cosmetic enhancements, the discipline encompasses much more. We distinguish between two primary branches: cosmetic surgery, aimed at enhancing appearance; and reconstructive surgery, intended to repair damage from injuries, birth defects, or medical conditions.

A JOURNEY THROUGH TIME

The history of plastic surgery is as old as civilization itself. The term 'plastic' comes from the Greek word 'plastikos,' meaning to mold or give form. Ancient Indian and Egyptian civilizations were known to practice simple forms of reconstructive surgery as far back as 2000 B.C.

The Renaissance period marked a significant turning point. In 16th century Italy, Gaspare Tagliacozzi, often referred to as the father of modern plastic surgery, developed methods to reconstruct noses, a procedure that would become the cornerstone of the field.

The World Wars also played a pivotal role, as the need to treat disfigured soldiers pushed innovations in reconstructive techniques. Sir Harold Gillies, a New Zealand-born surgeon, is celebrated for his contributions during this time, laying the groundwork for modern plastic surgery.

Today, plastic surgery is a rapidly evolving field, shaped by technological advancements and a growing understanding of human anatomy. From minimally invasive procedures to complex reconstructions, the scope of plastic surgery is vast.

This book is written for anyone curious about plastic surgery. Whether you are a medical student, a prospective patient, or simply interested in understanding this fascinating field, this book aims to provide a comprehensive overview. We will explore the technical aspects, the psychological motivations behind seeking surgery, and the ethical considerations that come with such powerful transformative capabilities.

In a world where appearance often drives perception, understanding the realities of plastic surgery is crucial. This book aims to dispel myths and provide a balanced view, acknowledging both the positive impacts and the potential risks and ethical dilemmas.

As we delve into the world of plastic surgery, we must also consider the ethical implications and the ever-changing public perception. From debates over elective surgeries in adolescents to the impact of media on body image, these topics warrant thoughtful discussion.

CHAPTER 2
EVOLUTION OF PLASTIC SURGERY

It's possible that humans have actively sought to better themselves since the dawn of time. It follows that the possibility that plastic surgery is among the oldest medical procedures in history should not be shocking. Over four thousand years of history are documented in the use of surgical techniques to treat facial injuries.

Skin grafting was the origin of plastic surgery in ancient India.

As early as 800 B.C., doctors in ancient India performed reconstructive surgery using skin transplants. Subsequently, plastic surgery progressed slowly in European nations. On the other hand, plastic surgery was more accepted in eastern medicine, and several cases of skin grafting and reconstructive surgery have been documented there throughout history.

Over the next few millennia, surgical procedures for plastic surgery, like the majority of medicine, advanced slowly as Indian techniques were brought to the West and later improved and repurposed for new uses. But during the Greco-Roman era, medical advancements were accomplished, and these advancements were recorded in antiquated writings that were eventually passed down across society.

Aulus Cornelius Celsus, a Roman physician, authored De Medicina during this time, which described surgical techniques for repairing noses, ears, and lips.2.Then, in the early Byzantine era, Oribasius created the Synagogue Medicae, a comprehensive medical encyclopedia. Several sections of this 70-volume opus were devoted to reconstructive methods for fixing face deformities.

The Renaissance

Even though reconstructive surgery was practiced during the early Middle Ages, the collapse of Rome and the advent of

Christianity prevented further substantial breakthroughs from occurring, bringing the field to a virtual standstill. Science was mostly replaced by mysticism and religion. In fact, during this period, the pope Innocent III proclaimed that Church law specifically forbade any sort of surgery.

Most of the time, the quest for scientific understanding has given way to an emphasis on deeper spiritual and human issues. Furthermore, the absence of requirements for sanitation and hygiene further jeopardized the safety of surgery patients. Nonetheless, a few small breakthroughs were achieved, such as the creation of a cleft lip repair technique in the ninth century.

More substantial scientific and technological developments during the Renaissance led to the creation of safer and more efficient surgical methods. Serafeddin Sabuncuoglu wrote an Islamic text named Imperial Surgery in the fifteenth century, which covers 191 surgical themes.3.

Bozkurt P, Babazade R, Salihoglu Z, and Basagaoglu I. The usage of Murkid, an anesthetic medication, by Serafeddin Sabuncuoğlu in the fifteenth century and its impact on the development of surgery. 2016 January.

Information about eyelid surgery and maxillofacial surgery is included. It also had a gynecomastia treatment program, which is thought to have served as the model for the current surgical breast reduction technique.

War Was the Source of Progress

Plastic surgery began to fall again in the seventeenth century, but by the end of the eighteenth century, the trend had reversed. But the next significant developments in plastic surgery wouldn't come about until the 20th century, when many troops needed reconstructive plastic surgery due to war-related injuries. In actuality, plastic surgery reached a new height in the medical community during World War I.

It was necessary for military physicians to treat numerous severe head and facial injuries brought on by contemporary weapons, the likes of which had not been seen before. These severe wounds required daring new advancements in reconstructive surgery techniques. Throughout and after the war, a number of Europe's most accomplished surgeons committed their careers to helping their nation's warriors return to full health.

This was actually the period when surgeons started to properly understand the impact that a person's outward look could have on their level of success in life. As a result of this realization, cosmetic surgery started to become recognized as a subspecialty of plastic surgery.

Surgeons are now able to conduct a bigger range of increasingly difficult surgeries because to advancements in anesthetic and infection prevention. These operations included the first known cases of operation that was purely "cosmetic," such as the first breast augmentation and rhinoplasty.

The American History of Plastic Surgery

Even though Europe was the birthplace of many of these groundbreaking medical advancements, the United States produced significant surgical advancements as well. In 1827, Dr. John Peter Mettauer performed the first cleft palate procedure in the history of medicine, employing surgical instruments he had designed himself. However, modern plastic surgery did not become acknowledged as a separate medical specialty until the beginning of the 20th century.

The Correction of Featural Imperfections, written by Dr. Charles Miller, was the first book specifically on cosmetic surgery when it was published in 1907. Despite being somewhat ahead of its time, many general surgeons condemned and labeled the material as "quackery."

Sadly, the medical establishment, which tended to see cosmetic surgeons in general—including Dr. Miller—as quacks or charlatans—shared this mindset.

During this period, Drs. William Luckett, Frederick Strange Kolle, and Vilray P. Blair were notable American surgeons. While Dr. Luckett reported a procedure for projecting ears in 1910 and Dr. Kolle published his work, Plastic and Cosmetic Surgery, a year later in 1911, Dr. Blair conducted the first closed ramisection of the jaw in 1909 and wrote Surgery and Diseases of the Mouth and Jaw in 1912.

The Value of an American Establishment

Johns Hopkins was one organization that made a significant contribution to the development and improvement of plastic surgery as well as surgery in general. It was there that America's first general surgery training program was established by Dr. William Stewart Halsted. His work, The Training of a Surgeon" published in 1904, served as the model for all contemporary surgical training programs. This would allow the United States to at last claim surgical expertise on par with that of Europe. The United States quickly started to outperform the other countries of the world, particularly in the area of surgical expertise.

Dr. John Staige Davis, widely regarded as the first American to focus exclusively on plastic surgery, also practiced at Johns Hopkins. The John Staige Davis Society of Maryland Plastic Surgeons. Our Maryland Society of Plastic Surgeons' past.

He devoted a significant amount of his life to creating specialized departments within the plastic surgery field. He once again emphasized the value of specialization within the discipline when he wrote a seminal piece for the Journal of the American Medical Association in 1916, describing the function of plastic surgery within the medical establishment.

1940s and 1950s

The time had obviously arrived in 1946 to launch a specialized scientific publication for plastic surgeons. The first volume of the Journal of Plastic and Reconstructive Surgery released its inaugural edition in July of that year. Since then, the publication has consistently provided a platform for the exchange of ideas and significant discoveries between plastic surgeons and other medical professionals, all with the goal of helping patients.

In 1950, the field of plastic surgery grew fully established in the medical establishment and started to gain public awareness thanks to the introduction of board certification and the publication of its own medical magazine. Further advancements in reconstructive surgery emerged from the Korean War field hospitals, such as the use of rotating flaps to treat severe skin abnormalities and injuries and internal wiring procedures to treat facial fractures.

CHAPTER 3
MODERN PLASTIC SURGERY

In the 1960s and 1970s, plastic surgery as we know it today truly began to take shape. During this time, there were also a lot of important scientific advancements. A recently developed material called silicone was becoming more and more well-known as an essential component of some plastic surgery operations. It was first applied to address skin blemishes. Then, in 1962, silicone was used to manufacture and introduce a novel breast implant device by Dr. Thomas Cronin. About ten years later, silicone implants were created for usage in every conceivable area of the body and face.

Plastic surgeons, such as Dr. Hal B. Jennings, who was named Surgeon General in 1969, and another who received a Nobel Prize, were rising to the top of the medical hierarchy.

Plastic surgery proponents and practitioners launched a major campaign to raise public knowledge and change the public's opinion of plastic surgery in the 1980s. The 1980s economic boom combined with an increase in consumer access to high-quality information started to make plastic and reconstructive surgery more widely available in America.

Despite issues brought on by the reform of healthcare, which resulted in substantial drops in insurance company reimbursement for reconstructive procedures, growth persisted into the 1990s. To remain in practice, many doctors were compelled to concentrate more on cosmetic procedures, and some chose to completely give up on reconstructive surgery.

Remarkably, a growing number of patients seemed to be pursuing cosmetic operations despite the mounting controversy around silicone breast implants. Then, in 1998, a bill requiring insurance companies to pay for post-mastectomy breast reconstruction surgeries was signed into law by President Bill Clinton.

Cosmetic surgery has seen a meteoric rise in popularity in the 2000s, and improvements in medicine have made restorative procedures accessible that were previously unattainable. The internet and television have joined the fast-paced communication age, allowing us to watch almost any type of plastic surgery treatment from the comfort of our homes.

The most significant development in plastic surgery right now is the shift toward less intrusive techniques intended to delay the appearance of aging. Indeed, the most common procedures performed nowadays use injectable materials like Botox and face wrinkle fillers. Over 1.1 million injections of Botox are reportedly given in the United States annually, and the figure is rising.

There has been a significant ethical discussion about the introduction of "Plastic Surgery Reality TV" particularly among plastic surgeons themselves. Despite its popularity, the television program Extreme Makeover was canceled in 2007 and has since generated some controversy. What kind of principles are we teaching with this kind of programming.

Naturally, Extreme Makeover has inspired a number of copycat series with plastic surgery themes. Undoubtedly, more people than ever before are pondering and discussing plastic surgery, even in spite of the continuous discussions regarding its benefits. The stigma traditionally associated with cosmetic surgery is disappearing, and as consumers, we are all better informed about the possible hazards and benefits of plastic surgery.

CHAPTER 4

TYPES OF PLASTIC SURGERY

Cosmetic surgery, aimed at improving appearance, has become increasingly popular. We explore common procedures, such as:

- **Facelifts and Neck Lifts**: Rejuvenating the face and neck area.

- **Breast Augmentation and Reduction**: Altering the size and shape of the breasts.

- **Rhinoplasty**: Reshaping the nose.

- **Liposuction**: Removing excess fat from various parts of the body.

- **Abdominoplasty (Tummy Tuck)**: Tightening abdominal muscles and removing excess skin and fat.

We'll also discuss less invasive procedures like Botox injections and dermal fillers, which have grown in popularity due to their accessibility and minimal downtime.

Facelifts and Neck Lifts

Overview

- **Purpose:** Facelifts (rhytidectomy) and neck lifts are surgical procedures aimed at rejuvenating the lower half of the face and neck. They address aging signs like sagging skin, deep creases, jowls, and loose skin on the neck.

- **Procedure:** The surgeon makes incisions typically along the hairline, extending around the ears. Excess skin is removed, underlying tissues are tightened, and the remaining skin is repositioned for a more youthful appearance. In a neck lift, similar techniques are used to tighten the skin and muscles of the neck.

Candidates for Surgery

Generally, good candidates are healthy individuals with noticeable signs of aging in the face and neck who have realistic expectations. Ideal candidates should also have good skin elasticity and bone structure.

Age Range most candidates are in their 40s to 70s, but there is no absolute age limit as long as the individual is healthy.

Procedure Details

Preparation: Involves a medical evaluation, possible adjustment of current medications, and avoidance of certain medications and supplements that can increase bleeding risk.

Anesthesia: Usually performed under general anesthesia or intravenous sedation.

Surgical Time It typically takes several hours, depending on the extent of the surgery.

Recovery Initial swelling and bruising are common, with most people returning to normal activities in 2 to 3 weeks. Full recovery and final results may take several months.

Possible Complications:

Common Risks: Include hematoma (blood collecting under the skin), infection, scarring, nerve injury leading to muscle weakness, and anesthesia risks.

Less Common Complications: May include prolonged swelling, skin loss, unsatisfactory results requiring additional surgery, and hair loss at the incision sites.

Postoperative Considerations:

- Patients are typically advised to keep their head elevated and avoid strenuous activities for several weeks. Follow-up appointments are crucial for monitoring healing and addressing any concerns.

Conclusion

Facelifts and neck lifts can significantly rejuvenate a person's appearance, but they are major surgical procedures. It's important for potential candidates to fully understand the risks, have realistic expectations, and choose a qualified, experienced plastic surgeon. As with any surgery, the benefits must be weighed against the potential complications and the individual's health and desired outcomes.

Breast Augmentation and Reduction

Breast Augmentation

This procedure involves enhancing the size and shape of the breasts using implants or fat transfer. It aims to increase fullness, improve symmetry, and restore breast volume lost after weight reduction or pregnancy.

Breast Reduction

This surgery reduces the size of large breasts, which can alleviate discomfort like back and neck pain, skin irritation, and posture problems. It involves removing excess breast fat, glandular tissue, and skin to achieve a breast size proportionate to the body.

Breast Augmentation Candidates

Ideal candidates are those looking to enhance breast size or symmetry. They should be physically healthy, have realistic expectations, and breasts must be fully developed.

Breast Reduction Candidates

Women experiencing physical discomfort or self-consciousness due to large breasts. They should be in good health, non-smokers, and without conditions that could impair healing.

Procedure Details

Breast Augmentation

Implants:

Silicone or saline implants are inserted through incisions made in inconspicuous areas to minimize visible scarring. The implant is placed either under the pectoral muscle or directly behind the breast tissue.

-Fat Transfer:

Fat is liposuctioned from other body parts and injected into the breasts. This option is for those seeking a moderate increase in breast size and more natural results.

Surgical Time:

Usually 1-2 hours.

Anesthesia

General anesthesia or intravenous sedation.

Breast Reduction

Procedure

Involves making incisions on the breasts, removing excess fat, glandular tissue, and skin, and then reshaping the remaining breast tissue. The nipple and areola may be repositioned to a more youthful height.

Surgical Time

Typically takes 2-5 hours.

Anesthesia

Usually performed under general anesthesia.

Possible Complications

Breast Augmentation Risks: Include implant leak or rupture, capsular contracture (scar tissue around the implant), changes in nipple or breast sensation, and irregularities in breast contour or shape.

Breast Reduction Risks

Include scarring, changes in breast or nipple sensation, potential inability to breastfeed, and, in rare cases, partial or total loss of the nipple or areola.

Recovery and Aftercare

Recovery Time:

Generally, it takes a few weeks to recover, with limitations on physical activities. Full healing may take several months.

Aftercare:

Involves wearing a support bra, managing pain with medication, and attending follow-up appointments to monitor healing.

Conclusion

Both breast augmentation and reduction surgeries can have profound psychological and physical benefits. However, they are significant procedures with associated risks and recovery times. Candidates should have a clear understanding of what the surgery entails, realistic expectations about the outcomes, and a qualified surgeon to ensure the best possible results.

Rhinoplasty

Reshaping the Centerpiece of the Face

Purpose

Rhinoplasty, commonly known as a nose job, is a surgical procedure to change the shape or improve the function of the nose. It can address aesthetic concerns such as size, shape, or symmetry, and functional issues like breathing difficulties.

Procedure: The surgery involves reshaping the bone and cartilage of the nose. This can include reducing the size, changing the angle, altering the tip, narrowing the nostrils, or correcting structural problems.

Ideal Candidates

Individuals looking to alter the appearance of their nose, improve breathing, or correct a birth defect or injury. Candidates should be in good overall health, non-smokers, and have realistic expectations about the outcome.

Age Considerations It's generally advised to wait until the nose has finished growing—around age 16 for girls and 17 for boys—before undergoing cosmetic rhinoplasty.

Procedure Details

Surgical Techniques: There are two main techniques:

Open Rhinoplasty: Involves an incision across the columella (the strip of tissue between the nostrils). This approach offers more visibility and control over nasal structures.

Closed Rhinoplasty: All incisions are inside the nostrils, resulting in no visible scarring. However, this method offers less access compared to the open technique.

Anesthesia

Typically performed under general anesthesia or local anesthesia with sedation.

Surgical Time: The procedure usually takes 1 to 3 hours.

Possible Complications

Common Risks: Include bleeding, infection, an adverse reaction to anesthesia, and breathing difficulties.

Aesthetic Complications: These can involve asymmetry, dissatisfaction with the appearance, and the need for revision surgery.

Other Risks: Scarring, a change in skin sensation, and persistent pain or swelling.

Recovery and Aftercare

Initial Recovery: Patients often experience swelling and bruising, especially around the eyes. A nasal splint is usually worn for the first week.

Activity Restrictions: Strenuous activities should be avoided for a few weeks.

Healing Time: While initial recovery may take a few weeks, it can take up to a year for the new nasal contour to fully refine.

Conclusion

Rhinoplasty can significantly alter one's appearance and improve nasal function, but it requires careful consideration due to its complexity and potential risks. Choosing a skilled and experienced surgeon, having realistic expectations, and adhering to postoperative care instructions are crucial for achieving the best results.

Liposuction

Sculpting the Body by Removing Unwanted Fat

Purpose

Liposuction is a surgical procedure designed to remove excess fat from specific areas of the body, such as the abdomen, hips, thighs, buttocks, arms, or neck. It's used to contour these areas and is not a means for significant weight loss.

Procedure: The surgery involves the use of a cannula (a thin, hollow tube) and a vacuum to suction fat from targeted areas. Various techniques, such as tumescent liposuction, ultrasound-assisted liposuction (UAL), or laser-assisted liposuction, might be used depending on the patient's needs and the surgeon's preference.

Ideal Candidates

Good candidates for liposuction are adults within 30% of their ideal weight who have firm, elastic skin and good muscle tone. It's essential for candidates to be healthy individuals without life-threatening illnesses or medical conditions that can impair healing.

Health and Lifestyle Considerations Non-smokers who have a positive outlook and specific goals in mind for body contouring are ideal candidates.

Procedure Details

Tumescent Liposuction:

Involves injecting a medicated solution into the fatty areas before the fat is removed, which can reduce pain and blood loss.

UAL: Uses sound waves to liquefy fat before it's suctioned out.

Laser-Assisted: Utilizes laser energy to liquefy fat.

Anesthesia: Can be performed under local anesthesia, intravenous sedation, or general anesthesia, depending on the extent of the procedure.

Surgical Time: Varies based on the amount of fat being removed and the number of areas treated, typically ranging from 1 to 4 hours.

Possible Complications

Common Risks: Include bruising, swelling, pain, numbness, or irritation in the treated areas, and fluid imbalance.

Surgical Risks: Can include infection, bleeding, uneven fat removal, or changes in skin sensation.

Serious Complications: Rare but can include deep vein thrombosis, cardiac and pulmonary complications, or persistent swelling.

Recovery and Aftercare

Initial Recovery: Patients typically experience swelling and discomfort for several days to weeks. Compression garments are often recommended to control swelling and shape the treated areas.

Activity Restrictions: Most people can return to work within a few days and resume normal activities within two weeks, although this varies based on the extent of the procedure.

Long-term Care: Results are usually long-lasting, provided the patient maintains a stable weight and follows a healthy lifestyle.

Conclusion

Liposuction can be an effective procedure for body contouring and removing stubborn fat deposits, but it's not a substitute for weight loss or a healthy lifestyle. Understanding the limitations and risks of the procedure is crucial for patient satisfaction. As always, the skill and experience of the surgeon play a vital role in the success of the procedure.

Abdominoplasty (TummyTuck):
Reshaping and Firming the Abdomen

Purpose:

Abdominoplasty, commonly known as a tummy tuck, is a surgical procedure that removes excess fat and skin and, in most cases, restores weakened or separated muscles in the abdominal area. This results in a smoother and firmer abdominal profile.

Procedure:

The surgery typically involves a horizontal incision in the area between the pubic hairline and belly button. The extent of the incision depends on the amount of excess skin. Once the abdominal skin is lifted, underlying weakened abdominal muscles are repaired. Excess fat and skin are then removed, and the remaining skin is sutured together.

Candidates for Surgery:

Ideal Candidates: Individuals with excess abdominal skin and fat that is resistant to diet and exercise. Ideal candidates are those in good physical health, at a stable weight, non-smokers, and with realistic expectations about the outcomes.

Not Recommended For:

Women planning future pregnancies (as vertical muscles in the abdomen that are tightened during surgery can separate again) and individuals who are planning significant weight loss.

Procedure Details:

Types of Tummy Tucks

Full Tummy Tuck: Addresses the entire abdominal area.

Mini Tummy Tuck: Focuses on the area below the belly button.

Anesthesia: Typically performed under general anesthesia.

Surgical Time: Can vary from 1 to 5 hours, depending on the complexity and extent of the surgery.

Possible Complications

Common Risks: Include swelling, bruising, discomfort, numbness, and fatigue.

Surgical Risks: Such as infection, bleeding, fluid accumulation (seroma), poor wound healing, and scars.

Other Complications: Include skin loss, blood clots, nerve damage, and risks associated with anesthesia. Asymmetry and unsatisfactory cosmetic results may require further surgery.

Recovery and Aftercare

Initial Recovery: Recovery time can vary, with most patients needing several weeks to a few months to recover fully. Drainage tubes may be placed under the skin to remove excess blood or fluid.

Activity Restrictions: Heavy lifting and strenuous activities should be avoided for several weeks. It's important to follow the surgeon's instructions on properly caring for the incision site and drains.

Long-term Outcomes: Results are generally long-lasting, especially if accompanied by a healthy lifestyle with proper diet and exercise.

Conclusion

An abdominoplasty can significantly improve the appearance of the abdomen, particularly in cases where diet and exercise alone have failed to achieve the desired results. However, it's a major surgery with a significant recovery period and potential risks. It's essential for patients to have a thorough understanding of the procedure, maintain realistic expectations, and choose a qualified, experienced surgeon for optimal results.

CHAPTER 5

THE PROCESS OF PLASTIC SURGERY

We delve into the comprehensive journey of undergoing plastic surgery, from the initial consultation to post-operative care and recovery. Understanding this process is crucial for anyone considering plastic surgery, as it involves careful planning, decision-making, and adherence to post-surgical care for the best outcomes.

Consultation and Decision-Making

Initial Consultation: The journey begins with an initial consultation, where patients meet with the plastic surgeon to discuss their goals and expectations. During this meeting, the surgeon evaluates the patient's medical history, current health status, and the specific area(s) to be addressed.

Setting Realistic Expectations: The surgeon explains what can realistically be achieved, discussing the benefits and risks associated with the procedure.

Visual Aids and Simulation: Many surgeons use photographs or computer simulations to show potential outcomes.

Decision-Making: Based on this information, patients can make an informed decision about whether to proceed with surgery. It's a time for patients to ask questions and express any concerns.

Pre-operative Preparations

Medical Evaluation: Includes lab tests and, in some cases, medical clearance from the patient's primary care physician or specialists.

Medications: Patients may be advised to adjust current medications, avoid certain over-the-counter drugs and supplements that can increase bleeding risk, and, in the case of smokers, strongly advised to stop smoking well in advance of surgery.

Preparation for Recovery: Patients are advised to arrange for someone to drive them home post-surgery and assist them for a few days if needed. Preparing a recovery area at home with essentials within easy reach is also recommended.

The Surgery Process

Admission: On the day of surgery, patients arrive at the surgical facility where they are prepped for the procedure.

Anesthesia: Administered based on the type and extent of the surgery. This could be local anesthesia with sedation, regional anesthesia, or general anesthesia.

The Procedure: The specifics of the procedure vary widely depending on the type of surgery being performed. It can range from minimally invasive procedures, taking an hour or less, to more complex surgeries requiring several hours.

Immediate Post-Operative Phase: After the surgery, patients are taken to a recovery area where they are closely monitored as they wake up from anesthesia.

Post-operative Care and Recovery

Immediate Post-operative Care: Involves managing pain, preventing infection, and monitoring for any signs of complications. Instructions on caring for incisions, drains, and prescribed medications are provided.

Follow-up Appointments: These are critical for monitoring healing and addressing any concerns. The first follow-up is usually within a week after surgery, with subsequent visits depending on the type of surgery and the patient's progress.

Recovery Time: Varies significantly based on the surgery. Some procedures allow a return to normal activities within days, while others require weeks or even months. Factors such as age, general health, type of surgery, and individual healing response all play a role in recovery time.

Long-term Care and Maintenance: Includes adhering to a healthy lifestyle, sun protection for surgical sites, and regular medical check-ups. The surgeon may provide specific instructions for scar care, exercise, and diet.

Conclusion

The process of plastic surgery is a comprehensive journey that requires informed decision-making, thorough preparation, and dedicated post-operative care. Each stage is critical in ensuring safety, minimizing risks, and achieving the desired outcomes. Understanding this process empowers patients to actively participate in their surgical journey, fostering a collaborative approach with their surgeon for the best possible results.

CHAPTER 6

PSYCHOLOGICAL ASPECTS OF PLASTIC SURGERY

The decision to undergo plastic surgery often extends beyond physical appearance, deeply intertwining with psychological factors. This chapter explores the psychological motivations behind seeking plastic surgery, its impact on self-esteem and mental health, and illustrates these aspects through relevant case studies.

Psychological Motivations for Surgery

Improving Self-Image: Many individuals turn to plastic surgery to improve their self-image. This desire can stem from dissatisfaction with a particular body part or a general feeling of not fitting into societal beauty norms.

Life Changes and Milestones: Significant life events, such as a major weight loss or childbirth, often motivate individuals to seek plastic surgery to restore or enhance their appearance.

Influence of Media and Society: The portrayal of idealized body images in media and social networks can significantly influence the decision to pursue cosmetic surgery.

Correcting Congenital or Acquired Deformities: For those born with congenital deformities or who have acquired deformities through accidents or disease, plastic surgery is often sought not just for aesthetic reasons but also for functional improvement and psychological relief.

Impact on Self-esteem and Mental Health

Positive Outcomes: Many patients report improved self-esteem and quality of life post-surgery, especially when the results align closely with pre-surgery expectations.

Risk of Unmet Expectations: If the surgical outcome doesn't meet a patient's expectations, it can lead to disappointment, depression, or even body dysmorphic disorder (BDD).

Body Dysmorphic Disorder: BDD is a mental health condition where a person obsessively focuses on perceived flaws in their appearance. Such individuals may seek multiple surgeries, often with little satisfaction.

Need for Psychological Evaluation: Some surgeons recommend psychological evaluation for patients who display signs of unrealistic expectations or mental health issues.

Case Studies

Case Study 1: A patient undergoes rhinoplasty to correct a perceived flaw in their nose. Post-surgery, they experience increased confidence and satisfaction, leading to improvements in social interactions and overall quality of life.

Case Study 2: A breast augmentation patient, despite a successful surgery, continues to feel dissatisfied with her body image, indicating underlying body dysmorphic disorder.

Case Study 3: A patient undergoing reconstructive surgery following an accident experiences not only physical restoration but also significant psychological healing, highlighting the multifaceted impact of plastic surgery.

Conclusion

The psychological aspects of plastic surgery are as significant as the physical ones. Understanding the motivations and potential mental health impacts is crucial for anyone considering plastic surgery. Surgeons and patients need to engage in open and honest discussions about expectations and potential psychological outcomes. A comprehensive approach, sometimes involving mental health professionals, can ensure that patients are making informed decisions and are prepared for the emotional as well as the physical aspects of their surgical journey.

CHAPTER 7
ETHICAL AND SOCIETAL CONSIDERATIONS IN PLASTIC SURGERY

This chapter explores the complex ethical and societal issues surrounding plastic surgery, acknowledging the significant influence of media and society on perceptions of beauty and the importance of regulatory and legal frameworks in maintaining standards in the field.

Ethical Dilemmas in Plastic Surgery

Balancing Desires with Medical Ethics: Plastic surgeons often grapple with ethical questions when patients' desires for aesthetic enhancement may not align with medical advisability. The decision to proceed with surgery must balance ethical considerations with respecting patient autonomy.

Body Dysmorphic Disorder (BDD): Ethical challenges arise when patients with BDD, a mental health disorder characterized by an obsessive focus on perceived physical flaws, seek cosmetic surgery. In such cases, ethical practice requires careful evaluation and, often, referral for psychological treatment rather than surgery.

Surgery in Minors: Cosmetic surgeries in minors, especially for non-medical reasons, raise ethical concerns. The patient's emotional maturity, informed consent, and the potential long-term impact of the surgery are critical factors to consider.

Commercialization and Ethics: The commercial aspects of plastic surgery, including marketing and promotion, can sometimes lead to ethical conflicts, particularly if they involve unrealistic promises or downplay the risks and recovery associated with procedures.

The Role of Media and Society in Shaping Attitudes

Media Influence: Media, including social networks, significantly shape societal attitudes towards beauty and, by extension, plastic surgery. This influence can create or reinforce unrealistic standards of beauty, impacting public perception and demand for cosmetic procedures.

Normalization vs. Stigmatization: While media exposure has normalized plastic surgery, making it more socially acceptable, it also risks stigmatizing individuals who choose not to or cannot afford these procedures.

Educational Responsibility: Media entities and influencers have a responsibility to provide accurate information about plastic surgery, highlighting both its potential benefits and risks. This can help form a more balanced and realistic public understanding of the field.

Regulatory and Legal Aspects

Regulatory Bodies and Standards: The plastic surgery field is governed by various regulatory bodies at both national and international levels. These organizations set standards for training, practice, and ethics in plastic surgery.

Legal Frameworks: Laws and regulations specific to medical practice and patient care apply to plastic surgery. These include guidelines on consent, patient privacy, and professional conduct.

Ensuring Safety and Quality: Regulations ensure that only qualified practitioners perform plastic surgery and that they adhere to the highest standards of patient care and safety.

Navigating Medical Malpractice: In cases of surgical errors or unmet patient expectations, the legal aspects of malpractice come into play. Understanding the legal ramifications and patient rights is crucial for both practitioners and patients.

Conclusion

Ethical and societal considerations are integral to the practice of plastic surgery. Understanding these aspects is crucial for practitioners to maintain professional integrity and for patients to make informed decisions. The media's role in shaping societal attitudes towards plastic surgery, coupled with robust regulatory and legal frameworks, ensures that the field evolves responsibly, prioritizing patient welfare and ethical practices.

CHAPTER 8

RISKS AND COMPLICATIONS IN PLASTIC SURGERY

In plastic surgery, as in all surgical fields, understanding and managing risks and complications is crucial. This chapter delves into the common risks associated with various plastic surgery procedures, strategies for managing complications, and the importance of patient education and informed consent.

Common Risks Associated with Surgery

Infection: Despite sterile techniques, infection remains a risk. Symptoms include redness, warmth, and unusual discharge at the surgical site.

Scarring: All surgeries leave scars, though plastic surgeons strive to minimize and conceal them. The severity of scarring varies based on the procedure and the patient's healing process.

Hematoma and Seroma: A hematoma is a pocket of blood, while a seroma is a pocket of serous fluid. Both can occur post-surgery, requiring drainage or additional procedures.

Nerve Damage: Some patients may experience temporary or permanent loss of sensation or muscle function in the operated area.

Anesthesia Risks: Anesthesia, while generally safe, carries risks like allergic reactions, respiratory issues, and, in rare cases, death.

Unsatisfactory Results: There's always a possibility that the outcome may not meet the patient's expectations, potentially necessitating revision surgeries.

Managing Complications

Early Detection: Regular post-operative check-ups are vital for early detection and management of complications.

Immediate Intervention: Some complications, like hematoma, may require immediate surgical intervention to prevent further issues.

Long-Term Management: For issues like scarring or minor asymmetries, long-term strategies, including silicone sheets, steroid injections, or laser treatments, may be employed.

Psychological Support: Addressing the psychological impact of complications is essential. Providing support and counseling can help patients cope with unexpected outcomes.

Patient Education and Informed Consent

Pre-Surgical Counseling: Prior to surgery, patients should be thoroughly informed about the procedure, including what to expect during recovery and potential risks and complications.

Informed Consent Process: Informed consent is more than a form; it's a process that ensures the patient understands the surgery's risks, benefits, alternatives, and potential outcomes.

Realistic Expectations: Surgeons should ensure that patients have realistic expectations. This includes discussing what the surgery can and cannot achieve.

Post-Surgical Instructions: Providing detailed post-surgical care instructions is crucial. This includes guidelines on wound care, activity restrictions, medication management, and signs of complications.

Conclusion

Understanding the risks and complications associated with plastic surgery is fundamental for both surgeons and patients. Effective management of these risks begins with a thorough pre-surgical evaluation and continues through post-operative care. Informed consent and patient education are key components in preparing for a surgical journey. By being well-informed, patients can make decisions that align with their goals and values, while surgeons can provide care that aligns with the highest standards of safety and ethics.

CHAPTER 9
PERSONAL STORIES AND INTERVIEWS

In this chapter, we delve into the human side of plastic surgery through interviews with surgeons and patients, exploring their experiences, narratives, and the psychological and social implications of these procedures. These personal stories provide valuable insights into the realities, challenges, and triumphs in the field of plastic surgery.

Interviews with Plastic Surgeons

Expert Insights: Interviews with seasoned plastic surgeons offer an inside look into the technical, ethical, and emotional aspects of performing surgeries. They share their motivations for choosing this field, the challenges they face, and the advancements they have witnessed.

Case Reflections: Surgeons reflect on memorable cases, discussing the decision-making process, surgical challenges, and the outcomes.

Ethical Considerations: These interviews also touch on how surgeons navigate ethical dilemmas, such as managing patient expectations, dealing with potential body dysmorphic disorder, and handling requests for unnecessary procedures.

Patient Experiences and Narratives

Diverse Patient Stories: This section includes narratives from patients who have undergone various types of plastic surgery, from cosmetic enhancements to reconstructive procedures.

Motivations and Expectations: Patients share their motivations for seeking surgery, their expectations, and how the reality of their outcomes aligned with these expectations.

Emotional Journey: These stories highlight the emotional journey that accompanies plastic surgery, including pre-surgery anxieties, post-surgery adjustments, and the impact on self-esteem and body image.

Psychological and Social Implications

Mental Health Impact: The chapter delves into how plastic surgery can affect mental health, both positively and negatively. It includes discussions on increased confidence and potential disappointments.

Social Perceptions and Changes: Patients discuss how their surgeries have affected their social interactions and relationships, shedding light on societal perceptions of plastic surgery.

Life Beyond Surgery: Narratives reveal how plastic surgery has impacted various aspects of patients' lives, including personal relationships, career, and overall lifestyle.

Conclusion

The personal stories and interviews in this chapter provide a multifaceted view of plastic surgery, highlighting the complexities and profound impacts of these procedures. By presenting a range of experiences from both surgeons and patients, this chapter offers readers a deeper, more empathetic understanding of the realities behind plastic surgery decisions, the emotional rollercoaster it can entail, and the profound impact it can have on individuals' lives.

CHAPTER 10
THE FUTURE OF PLASTIC SURGERY

This chapter explores the future of plastic surgery, focusing on emerging trends, evolving techniques, and the potential ethical and regulatory challenges ahead. It also discusses the anticipated developments in both cosmetic and reconstructive surgery, painting a picture of what the future may hold in this ever-evolving field.

Emerging Trends and Techniques

Technological Advancements: Advances in technology, such as 3D printing and laser techniques, are set to revolutionize the way surgeries are planned and executed. 3D printing, for example, could be used for creating customized implants or for precise pre-surgical planning.

Minimally Invasive Procedures: There is a growing trend towards minimally invasive or non-invasive procedures. Techniques such as laser therapy, cryolipolysis, and advanced injectables offer cosmetic enhancements with less risk and downtime than traditional surgery.

Regenerative Medicine: The field of regenerative medicine, including stem cell therapy and tissue engineering, is likely to have a significant impact on reconstructive surgery. This could potentially lead to more natural and effective restoration for patients who have suffered injuries or congenital defects.

Personalized Medicine: Advances in genetics and precision medicine may lead to more personalized approaches in plastic surgery, optimizing procedures based on individual genetic profiles.

Ethical and Regulatory Challenges Ahead

Managing Expectations with New Technologies: As new technologies emerge, managing patient expectations will become increasingly complex. There is a need for ethical guidelines to ensure patients are well-informed about the realistic outcomes of advanced procedures.

Regulatory Oversight of New Techniques: The introduction of new techniques and materials will require stringent regulatory oversight to ensure patient safety. This includes approval processes for new devices and products used in plastic surgery.

Global Disparities: As advanced techniques become more prevalent, there may be an increase in disparities in access to these technologies, raising questions about equity in healthcare.

The Future of Cosmetic and Reconstructive Surgery

Cosmetic Surgery: In cosmetic surgery, the future is likely to see a continued emphasis on natural and subtle results. Patients are increasingly seeking enhancements that do not drastically alter their appearance but rather refine and rejuvenate.

Reconstructive Surgery: The future of reconstructive surgery holds promise for more effective and life-changing procedures. With advancements in tissue engineering and regenerative medicine, reconstructive surgeries could offer results that closely mimic natural form and function.

Integration with Other Disciplines: The field of plastic surgery is likely to see increased collaboration with other disciplines, such as dermatology, oncology, and neurology, leading to more comprehensive care and innovative treatment approaches.

Conclusion

The future of plastic surgery is bright and full of potential, driven by technological innovations and a deeper understanding of human genetics and regenerative medicine. While this progress brings exciting possibilities, it also presents ethical and regulatory challenges that must be navigated carefully. The field must continue to evolve not just technologically but also ethically, ensuring that advancements benefit a broad range of patients while maintaining the highest standards of safety and care.

CHAPTER 11

CONCLUSION

This concluding chapter encapsulates the key points discussed throughout the book and reflects on the multifaceted impact of plastic surgery. It aims to provide a cohesive summary and final thoughts on the evolving field of plastic surgery, highlighting its complexities, advancements, and the profound effects it has on individuals and society.

Summary of Key Points

Scope and Evolution: We began by exploring the wide-ranging scope of plastic surgery, tracing its evolution from ancient practices to the sophisticated medical specialty it is today.

Types of Procedures: The diverse types of plastic surgery, from cosmetic enhancements like facelifts and breast augmentations to reconstructive surgeries addressing congenital defects or injuries, were examined to understand their purposes, techniques, and outcomes.

Surgical Process: We delved into the detailed process of plastic surgery, covering the stages from consultation and decision-making to the intricacies of the surgical procedures and the critical importance of post-operative care and recovery.

Psychological Impact: The psychological motivations for seeking plastic surgery and its significant impact on self-esteem and mental health were explored, supplemented by personal narratives and case studies.

Ethical and Societal Considerations: The ethical dilemmas, societal influences, and regulatory aspects associated with plastic surgery were discussed to understand the broader implications of these procedures.

Risks and Complications: Addressing the inherent risks and potential complications, the book emphasized the importance of patient education and informed consent in mitigating these issues.

Future Outlook: Looking ahead, we explored emerging trends, technological advancements, and the future challenges and opportunities in both cosmetic and reconstructive plastic surgery.

Final Thoughts on the Impact of Plastic Surgery

Transformative Power: Plastic surgery holds a unique and transformative power, capable of not only altering physical appearance but also impacting psychological well-being and quality of life.

Balancing Art and Science: The field represents a delicate balance between art and medical science, requiring a blend of technical skill, aesthetic judgment, and ethical consideration.

Patient-Centered Approach: Central to the practice of plastic surgery is a patient-centered approach, where understanding patient needs, managing expectations, and ensuring informed decision-making are paramount.

Continual Evolution and Ethical Responsibility: As the field continues to evolve with technological advancements, the responsibility to navigate these changes ethically and with patient safety in mind remains crucial. Surgeons, patients, and the broader medical community must work together to uphold these standards.

Global Impact and Accessibility: The impact of plastic surgery extends globally, transcending cultural and national boundaries. Efforts must continue to make these life-changing procedures accessible and equitable for all who need them, regardless of their geographic or socio-economic status.

Conclusion

Plastic surgery, in its many forms and complexities, is more than just a medical procedure. It's a journey that intertwines medical expertise with personal aspirations, ethical considerations, and societal influences. This book aimed to provide a comprehensive understanding of plastic surgery, shedding light on its many facets and the profound impact it has on individuals and society. As the field continues to advance and evolve, it remains a dynamic and integral part of the medical world, constantly reshaping our understanding of beauty, restoration, and the human body.